VASCULITIS DIET COOKBOOK:

FOR NEWLY DIAGNOSED

I0427261

Complete Beginner Procedures On Food Recipes, Guided Meal Plans, And Healthy Lifestyle Tips To Manage, Strive, And Live Well With Vasculitis

DR. EMMY BROOKS

ABOUT THIS BOOK

The "Vasculitis Diet Cookbook" stands as an indispensable guide for individuals navigating the complexities of Vasculitis, shedding light on the intricate relationship between diet and the management of this condition. The introductory section aptly sets the stage by emphasizing the paramount role of nutrition in dealing with Vasculitis, laying the foundation for the comprehensive exploration that follows.

Understanding Vasculitis becomes accessible through a thoughtful breakdown of its intricacies, types, and the profound impact it exerts on overall health. This knowledge is pivotal for readers seeking to take charge of their well-being. The subsequent section delves into the basics of a Vasculitis-friendly diet, elucidating the importance of specific nutrients tailored to alleviate the challenges posed by the condition.

The heart of the book lies in the practicality of implementation, with a detailed guide on meal planning, nutrient balancing, and the provision of sample meal plans catering to diverse dietary preferences. The incorporation of essential ingredients and nutrient-rich foods not only enriches the palate but empowers readers with a tangible tool for healthier living.

Navigating daily life is made more manageable with practical cooking tips and a collection of delicious yet health-conscious recipes. The inclusion of meal prep strategies, guidelines for dining out, and insights into managing special diets elevates this book beyond a mere cookbook, making it a comprehensive lifestyle companion for those grappling with Vasculitis.

Crucial lifestyle components such as exercise recommendations and stress management techniques are seamlessly integrated, emphasizing a holistic approach to Vasculitis management. Monitoring and adjusting one's diet is demystified, encouraging readers to maintain a vigilant yet sustainable connection with their nutritional choices.

The book's narrative gains additional depth through real-life success stories and inspirations, reinforcing the notion that a Vasculitis-friendly diet is not just a regimen but a transformative journey. The engaging and elevated tone throughout this invaluable guide ensures that readers embark on this journey with a sense of empowerment and optimism, fostering a commitment to a healthier and fulfilling lifestyle.

Copyright © 2023 by Dr. Emmy Brooks

All rights reserved. This book cannot be duplicated, saved, or sent in any way—electronic, mechanical, photocopying, recording, scanning, or otherwise—without the publisher's prior written consent, except for brief quotes used in reviews and certain other noncommercial uses allowed by copyright laws.

DISCLAIMER

This book's content is solely intended for general informative purposes. About the availability, applicability, correctness, completeness, and trustworthiness of the data or recipes in this book, the author provides no guarantees of any sort, either stated or implied. You bear full responsibility for any reliance you may have on such material.

The advice, diagnosis, or treatment provided by a qualified medical expert is not to be replaced by this cookbook. When in doubt about a medical problem, never hesitate to consult your doctor or another trained healthcare professional. Never ignore medical advice from professionals or put off getting it because of something you've read in this book.

At the time of publishing, the author of this book has taken reasonable steps to guarantee that the information is correct and current. He does not, however, guarantee that the data will be error-free or that it will satisfy any certain performance or quality standards. Any negative repercussions that may arise from using or applying the material in this book are not the responsibility of the author, publisher, or distributor.

In this book, references or mentions of individuals, products, websites, organizations, or other names are for informational purposes only and do not imply endorsement or affiliation with the author. The author has no control over the nature, content, and availability of referenced or mentioned entities. Any reliance on such information is at the reader's own risk.

The inclusion of any references does not necessarily imply a recommendation or endorse the views expressed within them. The author or publisher shall not be liable for any loss or damage arising out of or in connection with, the use of this book.

INTRODUCTION

Overview of Vasculitis:

To properly manage vasculitis, one must have a thorough understanding of the condition. The term "vasculitis" describes a collection of illnesses marked by blood vessel inflammation. Throughout the body, these blood vessels can be arteries, veins, or capillaries.

Depending on which organs and tissues are impacted, the inflammation may cause the blood vessels to weaken, narrow, or even scar. This can result in a variety of symptoms.

Let's start by dissecting the term "vasculitis." The letters "vascul" and "-itis" stand for blood vessels and inflammation, respectively. Thus, the term "vasculitis" refers to an inflammation of the blood vessels. When the body's immune system unintentionally targets its blood arteries, inflammation results, causing tissue damage and a range of symptoms.

Vasculitis comes in a variety of forms, from moderate to severe, and it can strike people at any age. While certain varieties can affect more than one organ at once, others mainly affect one or more organs, such as the skin, lungs, or kidneys. Although the precise origin of vasculitis is frequently unknown, infections, specific drugs, or other underlying medical disorders can occasionally cause it.

Vasculitis symptoms can differ significantly based on the blood vessels impacted and the degree of inflammation. Fatigue, fever, weight loss, joint and muscle discomfort, skin rashes, neurological issues, and organ dysfunction are typical symptoms. Vasculitis can be difficult to diagnose since its symptoms might resemble those of a wide range of other illnesses. A combination of medical history, physical examination, imaging studies, and blood testing may be needed.

After a diagnosis, drugs to lower inflammation and inhibit the immune system are usually used to treat vasculitis.

However, lifestyle choices like nutrition can also be important in controlling vasculitis and enhancing general health outcomes, in addition to medication therapy.

Diet is Crucial for Managing Vasculitis:

Because particular foods and nutrients can either assist reduce inflammation and promote healing or increase symptoms and induce flare-ups, diet plays a critical role in controlling vasculitis. Vasculitis cannot be cured by diet alone, but healthy eating choices can support medical interventions and enhance general health.

Inflammation reduction on all levels of the body is one of the main objectives of a vasculitis diet. Reducing inflammatory triggers in the diet can help minimize symptoms and lower the chance of problems because chronic inflammation is thought to be a major factor in the onset and progression of vasculitis.

A nutritious diet can also help maintain cardiovascular health in general and the immune system in particular, both of which are critical for those with vasculitis. Consuming a diet that is well-balanced and abundant in fruits, vegetables, whole grains, lean proteins, and healthy fats can supply vital vitamins, minerals, antioxidants, and other nutrients that lower oxidative stress, boost cardiovascular health, and enhance immune system function.

Moreover, several dietary ingredients have been connected to elevated inflammation and may make vasculitis symptoms worse in sufferers. Processed foods, refined carbohydrates, trans and saturated fats, and high sodium are a few of these. Individuals with vasculitis can assist reduce inflammation and improve symptom management by restricting or avoiding these inflammatory foods.

A vasculitis diet may emphasize supporting particular organs or systems impacted by the illness in addition to lowering inflammation. For instance, cutting back on sodium and avoiding foods that put stress on the kidneys, like processed meats and meals high in phosphorus, may help if renal vasculitis is present. In a similar vein, if the gastrointestinal tract is affected by vasculitis, avoiding potential triggers like spicy meals and caffeine and concentrating on easy-to-digest foods may help reduce symptoms.

Overall, it is impossible to exaggerate the role that nutrition plays in managing vasculitis. Individuals with vasculitis can minimize symptoms and lower their risk of consequences by following a nutrient-dense, anti-inflammatory diet customized to meet their specific needs and health objectives. Having strong collaboration with a physician or qualified dietitian can assist in guaranteeing that dietary guidelines are customized and successful in treating vasculitis.

CHAPTER ONE

INTRODUCTION TO VASCULITIS

A Concise Overview of Vasculitis

The rare and varied illnesses collectively known as "vasculitis" are typified by inflammation of the blood vessels. Small capillaries to massive arteries are among the blood vessels of different sizes that can be affected by inflammation. In vasculitis, the immune system—which normally defends the body against infections and illnesses—inadvertently targets blood vessels, causing swelling, constriction, and occasionally occlusion of the veins. Damage to tissues and organs may arise from this reduced blood flow.

As an autoimmune disease, vasculitis must be understood to determine its underlying causes. The immune system, which typically recognizes and attacks outside intruders, starts to target the body's tissues in autoimmune illnesses.

This immune reaction causes blood vessel irritation in the case of vasculitis. This autoimmune response may be brought on by a variety of factors, such as infections, genetics, or environmental exposure.

The type and location of the damaged blood vessels can have a significant impact on the symptoms of vasculitis. Depending on which organs are affected, common symptoms can include organ-specific symptoms, exhaustion, fever, weight loss, and pain in the muscles and joints. Timely diagnosis and treatment are essential to reduce complications and improve the quality of life for those who suffer from vasculitis.

Various Vasculitis Types:

Numerous kinds of vasculitis exist, each with distinct characteristics and affected regions. Vasculitis is a complicated and multifaceted illness. Giant Cell Arteritis (GCA) is one type that is frequently seen; it mostly affects the arteries in the head, particularly the temples. Another kind is called Polyarteritis Nodosa (PAN), and it affects multiple organs by inflaming medium-sized arteries.

Once known as Wegener's granulomatosis, granulomatosis with polyangiitis (GPA) is a kind of vasculitis that frequently affects the kidneys and respiratory system. Another variety that affects small blood vessels and can affect the kidneys and lungs is called microscopic polyangiitis (MPA). It is essential to identify the particular form of vasculitis to customize treatment plans.

Blood tests, imaging studies, and occasionally a biopsy of the afflicted tissue are all common components of diagnostic procedures. Immunosuppressive drugs may be part of treatment regimens after a diagnosis to control inflammation and stop more harm.

Vasculitis's Effect on General Health:

Vasculitis affects general health in a significant and diverse way. Because vasculitis is a chronic disorder, people with it may have emotional and psychological difficulties in addition to their physical symptoms.

Stress and worry might be exacerbated by the disease's uncertain course and the possibility of relapses.

Additionally, depending on the kind and intensity of the illness, vasculitis can affect particular organs and result in a variety of consequences. Renal failure, for example, might arise from kidney involvement, and cardiovascular issues can raise the risk of heart disease.

It is impossible to overestimate the significance of continuing medical care and early intervention in reducing the long-term effects on general health.

Diet and other lifestyle factors are becoming more widely acknowledged as important in the management of vasculitis. In addition to medicinal therapies, a well-planned diet can assist manage inflammation and promote general health. An anti-inflammatory diet, eating a balanced diet, and drinking plenty of water are all essential elements of a vasculitis-friendly way of living.

An all-encompassing strategy for managing vasculitis is crucial, as evidenced by the possible effects on organ function, mental health, and general quality of life. Individuals suffering from vasculitis can optimize their health and lessen the burden of this difficult condition on their everyday lives by attending to both the medical and lifestyle elements.

CHAPTER TWO

FOUNDATIONS OF A DIET FRIENDLY FOR VASCULITIS

The Role of Diet in the Management of Vasculitis

Vasculitis requires a multifaceted approach to management that extends beyond prescription medications. For those with vasculitis, nutrition is essential to maintaining their general health. A healthy, well-balanced diet that is supportive of vasculitis can help reduce symptoms, strengthen the immune system, and aid in the condition's overall treatment.

The effect that diet has on inflammation is one of the main reasons that it is essential for managing vasculitis. Blood vessel inflammation is a hallmark of vasculitis, and various foods can either reduce or increase this inflammatory response. For those with vasculitis, a diet high in anti-inflammatory foods can help lessen the intensity of their symptoms and improve their quality of life.

Furthermore, healthy eating strengthens the immune system, which is crucial for those with vasculitis. A compromised immune system might increase an individual's susceptibility to infections and exacerbate the symptoms of vasculitis. Therefore, for those who are controlling vasculitis, it becomes imperative to include immune-boosting elements in their diet.

Furthermore, nutrition is important in the management of various medical diseases like hypertension and cardiovascular problems that frequently accompany vasculitis. These coexisting diseases can benefit from a heart-healthy diet, which can enhance general health and well-being.

Comprehending the significance of diet in the management of vasculitis enables people to actively participate in their health. It offers a comprehensive approach to treatment, enhancing medical interventions and adding to a more thorough and successful approach to care.

Important Nutrients for People with Vasculitis:

1. Omega-3 Fatty Acids: Known for their anti-inflammatory qualities, omega-3 fatty acids can be found in walnuts, flaxseeds, and fatty fish. Including them in the diet can assist in reducing the inflammatory reaction associated with vasculitis. Supplements containing fish oil might be taken into consideration, but it's best to speak with a healthcare provider to figure out the right amount.

2. Antioxidants: Patients with vasculitis may benefit from a diet high in antioxidants. Antioxidants, included in fruits and vegetables, aid in the fight against inflammation and oxidative stress. Antioxidants can be found in abundance in kale, spinach, citrus fruits, and berries. A wide spectrum of antioxidants is ensured by including a variety of colored fruits and vegetables in regular meals.

3. Sources of Protein: The immune system and tissue healing both depend on protein. The diet should contain lean protein sources such as fish, chicken, lentils, and tofu. Consuming enough protein promotes general health and speeds up the healing process for those who have vasculitis.

4. Vitamin D: Vitamin D is important for healthy bones and the immune system. It's critical to make sure you're getting enough vitamin D because both vasculitis and its therapies may lower vitamin D levels. Natural sources include sunshine, fortified dairy products, and fatty fish; however, under a doctor's supervision, supplements can be required.

5. Whole Grains: Whole grains include vital minerals, fiber, and complex carbohydrates. Whole wheat products, quinoa, and brown rice are all excellent options. These foods offer a variety of nutrients that enhance general well-being, help maintain sustained energy levels, and support digestive health.

6. Hydration: People with vasculitis need to drink enough water, yet this is something that is frequently forgotten. Particularly during flare-ups, water helps to maintain blood volume and prevent dehydration.

Water-rich fruits and vegetables as well as herbal teas can help you stay hydrated overall.

7. Restricting Trigger items: People who have vasculitis should be aware of items that could worsen their symptoms as triggers. Processed foods, too much salt, and certain allergies are a few examples of them. Maintaining a meal journal can assist in pinpointing and removing particular triggers, leading to improved symptom management.

People can actively improve their health by concentrating on these essential nutrients and implementing a diet that is beneficial to those with vasculitis. A licensed dietician or other healthcare professional can offer individualized advice, ensuring that the food plan is in line with each person's preferences and health needs. Including these dietary adjustments can become a sustainable and successful aspect of managing vasculitis with a methodical and educated approach.

CHAPTER THREE

PLANNING YOUR MEALS

List of Helpful Substances:

1. Vibrantly colored fruits and veggies:

A diet that is friendly to vasculitis should include a wide range of vibrant fruits and vegetables. These colorful foods are full of vitamins, minerals, and antioxidants that improve general health and help lower inflammation. Try to fill your plate with as many different colors of vegetables as possible, such as berries, bell peppers, carrots, and leafy greens.

Start by choosing a couple of your favorites or ones that are easily found at your neighborhood grocery shop to make this step easier for beginners. Consider having spinach in your lunchtime salad, having blueberries for breakfast, and having sliced bell peppers as a snack.

Increase the variety of nutrients you eat by gradually experimenting with different options as you feel comfortable doing so.

2. Sources of Lean Protein:

Including lean protein in your diet is crucial for maintaining the health and regeneration of your muscles. Go for foods like fish, tofu, skinless chicken, and beans.

These meals offer a good source of protein without being overly heavy in saturated fats, which can aggravate inflammation. For starters, think about including baked fish, grilled chicken breast, or a basic lentil soup in your meals.

Start by switching out one or two sources of protein per week with lean alternatives. This methodical technique facilitates a smoother transition by allowing you to become used to new tastes and textures.

You will find fun ways to include these protein sources into your everyday routine as you experiment with different dishes.

3. Complete Grains:

Whole grains are an excellent source of fiber, important minerals, and complex carbohydrates. Make your choice from foods like oats, brown rice, quinoa, and whole wheat. These grains support healthy digestion and offer a steady supply of energy. Beginners might begin by switching to whole grains instead of refined grains. For example, replace white rice with brown rice or white bread with whole grain bread.

Proceed cautiously, incorporating one novel whole grain at a time, and progressively broaden your range of options. This guarantees that you locate options that fit your taste buds in addition to embracing healthier options. Try different cooking techniques and combine them with your preferred proteins and veggies to create a balanced dinner.

4. Good Fats:

For a balanced diet for vasculitis, it is essential to include sources of good fats. Add foods high in omega-3 fatty acids, like walnuts, flaxseeds, chia seeds, and fatty fish (salmon, mackerel). Vasculitis sufferers may benefit from these lipids' anti-inflammatory qualities. If you're a beginner, think about adding a plate of salmon to your weekly plan or topping your yogurt with chia seeds to start your day.

Replace processed foods' saturated fats with healthier fat substitutes over time. This may be picking a handful of almonds as a snack or using olive oil instead of butter. These minor changes over time can result in major enhancements to your diet as a whole.

5. Spices and Herbs:

By adding herbs and spices to your food, you can improve its flavor and get even more health advantages. Certain foods, like cinnamon, ginger, garlic, and turmeric, have anti-inflammatory qualities. Beginners might start by sprinkling a little turmeric into their soups or dressing salads with fresh herbs like cilantro or parsley.

Try a different herb or spice every week to progressively assemble a collection that goes well with your recipes. This gives your meals more diversity and incorporates more anti-inflammatory foods into your diet.

Foods High in Nutrients to Add to Your Daily Meals:

1. For breakfast:

Have a nutrient-rich breakfast to provide you with energy for the rest of the day. Think about alternatives like a bowl of overnight oats garnished with nuts and fruits, or a smoothie made with spinach, berries, and a dollop of protein powder. These options provide a good start to the day by providing a balance of vital nutrients in addition to excellent taste.

Beginners should make a fruit and yogurt parfait or have whole grain toast with avocado for breakfast. These healthy but simple options make a great start to the day without taking up too much time with elaborate meal prep.

2. Lunch:

A lunch that is friendly to vasculitis should include a variety of colorful veggies, healthy grains, and lean proteins. For those just starting, quinoa salad with mixed vegetables and grilled chicken or tofu is a simple yet wholesome option. A tasty and well-balanced dinner can be made with a whole-grain wrap filled with turkey, hummus, and crisp vegetables.

Make little progress by organizing your lunches ahead of time. Lunch prep can be streamlined by making a big batch of quinoa or marinating chicken on Sunday. In this manner, you'll develop the habit of progressively including nutrient-dense foods in your midday meals.

3. Dinner is

Dinner is a chance to produce healthful dishes and taste experiments. A straightforward but nutrient-dense dish is baked salmon with steamed broccoli and a side of roasted sweet potatoes. Beginners can also try vegetarian dishes like chickpea curry or lentil stew served over brown rice.

Simplify dinner preparations by becoming proficient in a few staple recipes. You can progressively broaden your cooking repertoire and include more vasculitis-friendly ingredients in your nightly meals as you gain more confidence in the kitchen.

4. Munchies:

Snacks high in nutrients are essential for sustaining energy levels during the day. Choose something like a handful of trail mix, a piece of fruit with almond butter, or Greek yogurt with a sprinkling of nuts. These snacks offer a mix of carbohydrates, healthy fats, and protein.

Invest in easy-to-grab snacks for beginners, such as pre-cut veggies with hummus or a tiny serving of mixed nuts. Making healthy decisions is made easier when these options are easily accessible, especially when things are hectic.

5. Drinking plenty of water

Although sometimes disregarded, enough hydration is essential to a diet for vasculitis. Water maintains general body functioning and aids in the removal of pollutants. Have a glass of water to start the day and try to have eight glasses or more during the day.

Herbal teas are another option if you want to increase your hydration levels and maybe reduce inflammation.

Establishing reminders and keeping a reusable water bottle on hand might help novices develop the habit of consistently staying hydrated. Try adding cucumber, lemon, or mint pieces to your infused water to give it a refreshing touch.

In summary, developing a diet that is compatible with vasculitis requires small, doable efforts. You may improve general health and efficiently control inflammation by adding these healthy elements to your meals and choosing nutrient-dense foods. Always keep in mind that the secret is to begin small, try different flavors, and progressively create a sustainable and pleasurable healthy eating regimen.

CHAPTER FOUR

CRUCIAL COMPONENTS OF A DIET FOR VASCULITIS
List of Helpful Ingredients

1. Foods that Reduce Inflammation:

Including anti-inflammatory items in your diet is essential for controlling the inflammatory response that comes with having vasculitis. Choose antioxidant-rich fruits and vegetables, like citrus fruits, leafy greens, and berries. These nutrients aid in lowering blood vessel inflammation and combating oxidative stress. Think about consuming a variety of vibrant veggies, such as bell peppers, broccoli, and carrots, as they offer a range of nutrients that support healthy blood vessels generally.

2. The Fatty Acids Omega-3:

The promotion of cardiovascular health and the reduction of inflammation are two major functions of omega-3 fatty acids. Consume fatty fish, such as mackerel, sardines, and salmon, as they are great providers of these healthful fats. If you're not a fan of seafood, you may still include foods like flaxseeds, chia seeds, and walnuts in your diet to help manage your vasculitis because they also contain omega-3 fatty acids.

3. Complete Grains:

To improve the nutritional composition of your meals, switch out processed grains for whole grains. Whole grains include important vitamins, minerals, and fiber. Examples of these are quinoa, brown rice, and oats. Fiber promotes overall cardiovascular health by assisting with digestion and helping to keep blood sugar levels steady. To ensure a smooth and sustainable transition, begin as a novice and gradually replace refined grains with their whole counterparts in your favorite recipes.

4. Trim Proteins:

To maintain the health of your muscles and reduce your intake of saturated fat, use lean protein sources. Lean meats, tofu, skinless chicken, and lentils are also great options. These proteins supply necessary amino acids and aid in tissue repair without adding extra fat, which may exacerbate inflammation. Try easy cooking techniques such as baking, grilling, or steaming to keep these protein sources' nutritious content intact.

5. Spices and Herbs:

Make use of the anti-inflammatory qualities of herbs and spices. Spices like cinnamon, ginger, garlic, and turmeric can be useful additions to your kitchen toolkit. These nutrients help lower inflammation in addition to improving the flavor of your food. If you're a beginner, begin by adding these spices to well-known recipes and progressively increasing their amount until they suit your taste buds.

Foods High in Nutrients to Add to Your Daily Meals

1. Vibrantly colored fruits and veggies:

Try to load your plate with as many different hues of fruits and veggies as possible. These colorful foods are high in antioxidants, vitamins, and minerals that promote general health. Make aesthetically pleasing salads or add fruits to smoothies for a delicious and nourishing approach to have your daily needs met. To progressively broaden your palette as a beginning, concentrate on trying one or two different fruits or vegetables per week.

2. Good Fats:

To support cardiovascular health, embrace sources of healthy fats including avocados, almonds, and olive oil. These fats add to a feeling of fullness and supply vital nutrients. Try putting slices of avocado on sandwiches or mixing some almonds into your yogurt in the morning. These modest adjustments can have a big effect on your daily nutrient intake and help you manage your vasculitis.

3. Low-fat dairy products or dairy substitutes:

To guarantee sufficient consumption of calcium, opt for low-fat dairy products or fortified dairy substitutes such as soy or almond milk. Calcium is essential for healthy bones, and people with vasculitis in particular need to preserve their bone density. Start by gradually replacing your standard dairy products with their reduced-fat equivalents to reduce your consumption of saturated fat while still fulfilling your nutritional requirements.

4. Variety of Lean Protein Sources:

Lean protein foods including fish, poultry, tofu, and beans will help you diversify your protein intake. This type guarantees a balanced consumption of vital amino acids free of too much-saturated fat. Try varying the sources of protein in your meals; for example, try a new fish recipe or look into plant-based protein options. This methodical technique guarantees a well-balanced nutrient profile and lets you choose satisfying substitutes.

5. Whole Grains and Foods High in Fiber:

Give priority to foods high in fiber and whole grains to maintain stable energy levels and promote digestive health. To begin, replace refined grains in staple foods like pasta, rice, and bread with whole grain substitutes. Your digestive system will adjust more easily to this gradual shift, and for added nutritional value, try quinoa, bulgur, and barley, among other whole grains.

Optimal health and well-being can be achieved by implementing a gradual and sustainable strategy to adjust to a vasculitis-friendly diet by incorporating these healthy nutrients and nutrient-rich foods into your daily meals.

CHAPTER FIVE

PRACTICAL COOKING TIPS

Cooking Methods Suitable for Vasculitis Patients:

When writing a cookbook specifically for people with vasculitis, it's important to think about culinary techniques that improve flavor while also being good for your health. Choosing cooking methods that maintain the nutritional value of ingredients is essential for those who are taking care of vasculitis. Let's look at a few cooking techniques that support vasculitis patients' nutritional requirements.

1. **Steaming:** This mild cooking technique helps food keep as much of its nutrients as possible. It is cooking food without immersing it in water using steam. This technique works especially well for veggies because it stops leaching, which loss of nutrients. Buy a good steamer or construct a temporary one by setting a metal colander over a

pot of simmering water to add steam to your vasculitis-friendly recipes. To retain flavor and nutrients, steam seafood, poultry, or vegetables until they are soft.

2. Poaching: Cooking food by slowly boiling it in a liquid—typically broth or water—is known as poaching. For fragile proteins like fish and eggs, this technique works perfectly. To poach, bring the ingredients to a gentle simmer rather than a rolling boil so they cook gradually and uniformly. Poaching is a good alternative for patients with vasculitis because it keeps moisture in and minimizes excessive nutrient loss. Try poached eggs or seafood to spice up your cookbook without sacrificing the delicate cooking method.

3. Baking: Baking is an adaptable technique that lets you make tasty food without using a lot of butter or oil. It works particularly well when cooking lean foods like turkey or chicken. Marinate ingredients with herbs and spices to add flavor without adding too much sugar or salt and preserve nutrients. Another baking alternative is to roast vegetables in the oven, which retains nutritional integrity while caramelizing natural sugars and enhancing flavors.

4. Grilling: Without adding extra fat, grilling gives food a smokey, charred flavor. Select lean pieces of meat or poultry and marinate them with herbs and spices to improve the flavor while grilling for vasculitis patients. Vegetables grilled on a grill add flavor and support a diet high in nutrients. Precook meats partially before grilling to prevent charring and help limit the production of potentially hazardous chemicals.

5. Sauteing is the process of swiftly frying food over medium-high heat in a tiny amount of oil. Although it might not be the main treatment for people with vasculitis, it can be applied in moderation. To preserve the nutritional value, use heart-healthy oils like olive oil and cook them for a short period. For some extra diversity in your cookbook, try this approach for gently cooking small servings of protein or vegetables.

These techniques when combined into a cookbook catering to those with vasculitis guarantee that people can eat a wide variety of tasty dishes without sacrificing the nutritional value needed to manage their disease.

How to Keep Nutrients Safe During Cooking:

When creating a cookbook for the vasculitis diet, maintaining the nutritional content of the products is crucial. Take into account the following suggestions to preserve nutrient content while cooking to guarantee the best possible health outcomes for individuals with vasculitis.

1. Reduce Water Usage: Try to use as little water as possible when cooking, particularly when blanching or boiling vegetables. Nutrient leaching can occur by using too much water. For maximum retention of any nutrients that are soluble in water, use steam or very little water, and think about adding the cooking liquid to the dish.

2. Select Fresh Ingredients: Whenever feasible, go for seasonal, fresh produce. When it comes to nutrients, fresh products frequently have higher levels than processed or frozen ones. A varied spectrum of vitamins and minerals can be found in your meals if you choose a range of vibrant fruits and vegetables.

3. Reduce the amount of time that passes between food preparation and cooking to minimize nutritional exposure to light and air. To maintain the highest nutritional content, opt for rapid and effective cooking techniques. Quick cooking techniques that help preserve nutrients in vegetables and meats include stir-frying and flash-cooking in a hot oven.

4. Use Nutrient-Rich Cooking Liquids: When cooking with liquids, choose nutrient-rich options such as low-sodium vegetable stocks or homemade broths. This gives the food flavor and provides the necessary vitamins and minerals. Steer clear of using processed or high-sodium broths excessively to keep your heart healthy.

5. Incorporate Raw or Lightly Cooked Ingredients: To optimize nutrient consumption, incorporate raw or lightly cooked ingredients into your dishes. Think about mixing raw veggies into salads or finishing recipes with fresh greens and herbs. This guarantees that certain nutrients are not cooked while also adding a sudden burst of freshness.

6. Maintain Vitamins with Appropriate Storage: Preservation of nutrients begins even before cooking. To preserve their vitamin content, refrigerate fruits and vegetables in the refrigerator or a cool, dark spot. Pay attention to how long you store food to avoid spoiling and nutrient loss.

7. Select Heart-Healthy Fats: When using oils or fats in cooking, use heart-healthy varieties such as avocado or olive oil. These oils contribute to the dish's overall nutritional profile in addition to enhancing flavors. To support cardiovascular health, usage of saturated and trans fats should be minimized.

These suggestions, when added to your cookbook on the vasculitis diet, will guarantee that people may eat tasty, nutrient-dense meals that meet their nutritional requirements and help them manage their disease.

CHAPTER SIX

APPETIZING AND HEALTHFUL RECIPES

Easy Recipes For People With Vasculitis

Yes, let's go to work creating easy, tasty, and nourishing foods just for those who are taking care of their disease. In creating recipes for this use, it is important to balance the nutritional value with the flavor. These recipes aim to tantalize the senses while cooking with mindfulness and nutrient-dense ingredients to improve overall well-being.

Quinoa Breakfast Bowl For Breakfast

1. Step 1: Assemble Your Ingredients: Start by putting your ingredients together. Quinoa, eggs, avocado, fresh veggies (such spinach, cherry

tomatoes, and bell peppers), and your preferred seasonings—like salt, pepper, and a dash of nutritional yeast for flavor—are the ingredients for this filling breakfast bowl.

2. Step 2: Prepare the Quinoa: To get rid of any bitterness, rinse the quinoa in cold water. Then, using a 1-part quinoa to 2-parts water ratio, mix it with water in a pot. Once it reaches a boil, lower the heat and simmer the quinoa for around fifteen minutes, or until it becomes fluffy and the water has been absorbed.

3. Step 3: Sauté the Vegetables: Chop your veggies as the quinoa cooks. One tablespoon of olive oil should be heated over medium heat in a skillet. Add the vegetables and sauté for 5 to 7 minutes, or until they are soft but have retained their color. For extra taste, lightly season them with salt and pepper.

4. Step 4: fry the Eggs: Crack the eggs and fry them in the same skillet until they are the desired doneness. You can cook them to get a crispy edge or scramble them for a softer texture.

5. Step 5: Assemble Your Bowl: Now that everything is prepared, put your breakfast bowl together. Place a heaping portion of cooked quinoa on the bottom, then add your cooked eggs, sliced avocado, and the sautéed vegetables on top. If desired, top with nutritional yeast for an extra burst of cheesy flavor.

6. Step 6: Savor Your Nutrient-Packed Breakfast: At this point, you may start enjoying your quinoa breakfast bowl. Its rainbow of brilliant hues not only makes it visually appealing, but it's also nutrient-rich food that will power your day. While vegetables give a variety of vitamins and minerals to support general health, quinoa offers a substantial amount of protein and fiber.

Mediterranean Chickpea Salad For Lunch

1. Step 1: Gather Your Ingredients: To make this light and filling lunch choice, gather cucumber, cherry tomatoes, red onion, feta cheese

(optional), fresh parsley, lemon juice, olive oil, salt, and pepper along with canned or cooked dried chickpeas.

2. Step 2: Ready the Chickpeas: Give them a good rinse and drain if you're using canned chickpeas. If you're making them from scratch, soak them in water overnight and simmer until they get soft. Before utilizing them in the salad, let them cool.

3. Step 3: Chop Your Vegetables: Finely chop the fresh parsley, thinly slice the red onion, chop the cucumber, and cut the cherry tomatoes in half. For the salad to be evenly distributed, you want all the ingredients to be around the same size.

4. Step 4: Put the salad together: Put the chopped veggies, crumbled feta cheese (if using), chickpeas, and Kalamata olives in a big mixing bowl. After adding a drizzle of lemon juice and olive oil, taste and add salt and pepper as needed. Mix everything until thoroughly incorporated.

5. Step 5: Allow the Flavors to Marinate: After assembling the salad, set it aside for a few

minutes so that the flavors can combine. To make sure that every bite is brimming with deliciousness inspired by the Mediterranean, this step is essential.

6. Step 6: Present and Savor: Your salad of Mediterranean chickpeas is now prepared for serving! Enjoy it as a healthy and wholesome lunch choice by dividing it into individual portions. This dish, which combines crunchy veggies, zesty feta cheese, and protein-packed chickpeas, will fill you up and give you energy for the rest of the day.

The Supper Will Be Baked Salmon And Roasted Veggies.

1. Step 1: Gather Your Ingredients: To make this tasty supper choice, you'll need olive oil, garlic, lemon, fresh herbs (like thyme or rosemary), salt, pepper, and fresh salmon fillets. You may also use a variety of veggies, such as broccoli, carrots, and red bell peppers.

2. Step 2: Get the Salmon Ready: Set the oven to 400°F, or 200°C. Arrange the salmon fillets onto a parchment paper-lined baking sheet. Olive oil and freshly squeezed lemon juice should be drizzled over them. Season with salt, pepper, chopped herbs, and minced garlic.

3. Step 3: Prepare the Vegetables: Cut up your veggies as the oven heats up. Cut them into little pieces, then place them on a different baking sheet. Add a drizzle of olive oil and season with pepper and salt.

4. Step 4: Bake Everything at Once: Preheat the oven and add the prepared vegetables and the seasoned fish to it. Bake for 15 to 20 minutes, or until the veggies are soft and have a hint of caramelization and the salmon is cooked through and flakes readily with a fork.

5. Step 5: Plate and Serve: Take everything out of the oven once it's perfectly cooked. Arrange the roasted veggies and baked salmon on individual plates, and feel free to add more fresh herbs as a

garnish. Serve this healthy dinner meal hot and savor its delicious flavors and textures.

Even inexperienced cooks can produce tasty and nourishing meals that are customized to benefit vasculitis patients by following these easy-to-follow instructions. It's simple to incorporate each recipe into a balanced diet because it emphasizes both flavor and health advantages.

These recipes will not only fuel your body but also delight your taste senses. Try them for breakfast (quinoa bowl), lunch (a cool Mediterranean chickpea salad), or dinner (a savory baked salmon with roasted veggies).

CHAPTER SEVEN

TECHNIQUES FOR PREPARING MEALS

Time-saving Methods for Preparing Meals:

Time-saving strategies are crucial to ensuring an effective and long-lasting meal prep procedure while starting a Vasculitis diet. Starting with a well-thought-out plan is crucial for beginners. Choose a collection of dishes to start that follow the Vasculitis dietary recommendations. These dishes have to include anti-inflammatory components and be easy enough for a novice to prepare.

Consider creating a weekly food plan to save time. This simplifies the cooking process and aids in food purchasing organization. Select recipes that call for similar ingredients to reduce the amount of food you have to buy and cut. When making your grocery list, go for fresh, whole foods like fruits, vegetables, lean meats, and whole grains that are high in antioxidants and anti-inflammatory qualities.

Set aside some time in advance to wash, chop, and portion your ingredients. This makes sure that everything is ready to cook when the time comes during the week, and that cooking itself becomes easier. If you want to speed up this process even further, think about utilizing appliances like a food processor or already-chopped veggies.

For beginners, using time-saving kitchen appliances can be a game-changer. Instant pots, air fryers, and slow cookers are a few examples of appliances that can drastically cut down on cooking time without sacrificing the nutritional value of the food. Another useful method is batch cooking, which involves making bigger batches of a certain dish and dividing it into manageable parts for the week. This way you have a choice of dishes to pick from and only have to cook a few times.

Lastly, plan out the sequence in which you prepare your meals. Start with recipes that can simmer while you work on other items or that call for lengthier cooking periods. By doing this, you may make the most of your time in the kitchen while still cooking scrumptious and nutritious meals that fit your Vasculitis diet.

Options for Batch Cooking and Freezing:

A key component of a good meal prep is batch cooking, particularly for people following a Vasculitis diet. It entails cooking more food all at once, giving you a stockpile of meals that are ready to consume all week long. This procedure can be intimidating to beginners, but with a methodical approach, it becomes a pleasant and simple chore.

Start by choosing recipes that work well in large quantities. The best recipes are those that freeze well and reheat without losing flavor or texture. Think of filling casseroles, soups, stews, and salads made with grains. Not only are these meals practical, but they also enable a varied and well-balanced diet.

Make a thorough shopping list based on the ingredients needed for each recipe after you've selected your favorites. Buy fresh, high-quality produce and lean meats that meet the nutritional requirements of those with vasculitis. When you're ready to prepare, schedule a specific period, preferably over the weekend, to devote yourself to batch cooking.

Before you begin cooking, prepare all of the ingredients methodically. Prepare the spices and herbs ahead of time, chop the veggies, and marinate the proteins. This guarantees a seamless and effective cooking experience, particularly for beginners who might still be honing their cooking techniques.

Consider serving quantities as you begin to cook. Separate the cooked foods into bite-sized portions so that it will always be simple to get a well-balanced meal when needed. Invest in freezer-safe, high-quality storage containers to preserve the flavor and freshness of your batch-cooked meals.

An essential part of batch cooking is freezing. Before placing the prepared meals in the freezer, let them cool fully.

For ease of identification, write the dish's name and preparation date on the label of each container. This keeps track of your frozen inventory and guarantees that you eat the meals in a fair amount of time.

To enjoy a dinner that has been batch prepared, either thaw it overnight in the fridge or reheat it straight from frozen, making sure to follow the recipe instructions for each dish. This method of preparing meals in bulk and freezing them not only saves time throughout the workweek but also guarantees that you always have a selection of meals that are suitable for people with Vasculitis.

SECTION EIGHT

DINING OUT WHILE HAVING VASCULITIS

Rules Regarding Eating Out
Making Knowledgeable Decisions at Restaurants

Following a specific diet is essential for controlling symptoms and enhancing general health when managing vasculitis. Eating out might be difficult, but it can be made more tolerable with the correct rules. Making educated decisions at restaurants requires proactive planning and forward thinking. This is a detailed guide to assist you manage eating out while you have vasculitis.

1. Investigate and Choose Restaurants Carefully:

Start by looking up local eateries that have menu items that fit within a vasculitis-friendly diet. These days, a lot of eateries publish nutritional information on their websites, which makes it simpler to find healthy options. Choose restaurants with a varied menu so you can find more options that fit your dietary requirements.

2. Make a Plan:

Spend some time looking over the online menu before you go to the restaurant. This enables you to plan your lunch and evaluate the possibilities available with care. Seek for dishes that feature a range of vibrant veggies, nutritious grains, and lean proteins. Steer clear of processed foods, high-salt foods, and fats that are saturated since they can aggravate vasculitis-related inflammation.

3. Explain Dietary Limitations:

When you get to the restaurant, make sure the server knows about any dietary requirements you have. It's critical to be specific about your requirements, such as staying away from particular components or cooking techniques. Vasculitis sufferers can dine in safety because most restaurants are willing to comply with particular dietary requests.

4. Select Whole Grains and Lean Proteins:

Choose lean protein options such as fish, tofu, or grilled chicken for your main dish. To ensure that your meal is well-balanced and nutrient-rich, serve it with full grains like brown rice, quinoa, or whole wheat pasta. These options supply vital nutrition without inducing vasculitis-related inflammation.

5. Accept Vibrant Vegetables:

A range of vitamins and antioxidants can be added to your meal in addition to flavor by including a choice of colored veggies. If you want to keep the dish healthful and low in inflammation, go for sautéed or steamed veggies instead of fried ones.

6. Take Care with Sauces and Dressings:

Preservatives, hidden sugars, and other unwanted components can be found in the sauces and dressings served with a lot of restaurant foods. To help you manage how much you eat, ask for dressings and sauces on the side. As an alternative, ask for healthier options or just basic olive oil and vinegar to enhance the flavor.

7. Control of Portion:

Food quantities at restaurants are frequently bigger than necessary, which can cause overindulgence. To prevent consuming too many calories, think about splitting an entree with a dining partner or request a half serving. Portion control is crucial for maintaining a healthy weight and general well-being, particularly for those who have vasculitis.

8. Maintain Hydration with Nutritious Drink Options:

Selecting food items is not as important as choosing the correct beverages. Choose low-sugar beverages like water, herbal tea, or other drinks to stay hydrated without adding extra calories or chemicals. Steer clear of excessive caffeine and sugar-filled beverages as these may exacerbate inflammation.

9. Conscious Eating Techniques:

Savor each bite and be aware of your body's signals of hunger and fullness to engage in mindful eating. By allowing your body to signal when it is full, eating slowly helps to maintain healthy digestive tract function and avoid overindulging. Eating in a relaxed and pleasurable way has a great effect on your general health.

10. Sweets and Treats:

Although moderation is key, exercise caution when selecting desserts. To fulfill your sweet desire without straying from your vasculitis-friendly diet, think about splitting a dessert with friends or going for a fruit-based option. Recall that moderation is essential, and making thoughtful decisions makes eating out more pleasurable and health-conscious.

Vasculitis sufferers can comfortably manage eating out by following these doable steps and making well-informed decisions that support their nutritional needs and general well-being.

CHAPTER NINE

HANDLING SPECIAL DIETS

Dairy-free, gluten-free, and Additional Dietary Concerns:

For those with vasculitis, following a gluten- and dairy-free diet is essential since certain foods might aggravate inflammation and provoke immunological reactions. Learning about substitute components that are safe to eat is the first step in managing these dietary concerns. Replace gluten (a protein present in wheat, barley, and rye) with gluten-free flour like rice flour, coconut flour, or almond flour. Non-dairy substitutes such as almond milk, coconut milk, or oat milk can be used in place of dairy products. Because processed foods may include concealed dairy or gluten levels, it's critical to carefully check food labels.

The key to negotiating dairy- and gluten-free diets is meal preparation. To ensure a stress-free and efficient grocery shopping experience, start by compiling a list of foods that are safe and harmful. Choose items that are naturally free of gluten and dairy, such as fruits, vegetables, lean meats, and gluten-free grains like rice or quinoa. By trying out several recipes and progressively developing a repertoire of tasty, safe meals, people will gain the confidence to effectively manage their nutritional needs.

Think about working with a dietitian or nutritionist to develop a customized meal plan based on nutritional needs. They can offer insightful information on guaranteeing sufficient nutrient intake and averting possible dangers. In addition, participating in internet forums or support groups devoted to dietary restrictions and vasculitis can provide a plethora of helpful advice and experiences from those with similar conditions, creating a supportive environment.

Patience is essential when negotiating a gluten-free and dairy-free lifestyle as a beginner. It may seem intimidating at first to learn how to read food labels, spot hidden allergies, and try out new recipes. But with patience and effort, anyone can learn how to cook without using gluten or dairy, which makes it a sustainable and fun aspect of managing vasculitis.

Recipe Modification for Certain Dietary Requirements:

The ability to modify meals to meet particular dietary requirements can significantly improve the quality of life for those who have vasculitis. The procedure entails replacing potentially inflammatory chemicals with healthy, safe substitutes. Knowing each ingredient's function in a recipe and finding appropriate substitutes is one of the most important factors to take into account.

When modifying recipes, begin by concentrating on the essential elements of a meal. For instance, flour is a basic ingredient in baking and frequently contains gluten. Try substituting gluten-free flour such as rice, coconut, or almond flour. Similar to dairy, consider non-dairy substitutes like soy, coconut, or almond milk to keep the flavor and consistency you want in a variety of dishes.

It is important to approach recipe adaptation with imagination and receptivity. Understand that some recipes call for more than one substitution and that not all substitutions are equally effective in all situations. Recording your successful modifications in a journal and noting the particular materials you used might be a useful tool for future culinary adventures.

Consider dissecting a favorite recipe, ingredient by ingredient, as a useful step-by-step recipe book. Look into and choose appropriate replacements for every ingredient, making sure they comply with nutritional guidelines. Introduce modifications gradually, taste-test the results, and make necessary adjustments to quantities or try other options until you get the desired result.

Make use of cookbooks and internet resources that are dedicated to gluten- and dairy-free cooking. These frequently include well-tested recipes and practical advice for a successful adaption.

Furthermore, consulting with seasoned chefs in the vasculitis community might provide insightful advice on successful dish alterations.

To sum up, customizing recipes to fit particular dietary requirements is a powerful ability that lets people with disabilities prioritize their health while still enjoying a wide variety of delicious meals. With trial and error, investigation, and an open mind to new ingredients, even beginners may learn to adapt recipes to meet their specific dietary needs.

CHAPTER TEN

VITAMINS AND SUPPLEMENTS

Recognizing Supplements' Functions:

It's critical to understand the critical function supplements play in promoting general health and reducing the effects of the condition when controlling Vasculitis with a customized diet. An inflammation of the blood vessels known as vasculitis can have a major impact on the immune system and the general health of the organs. This emphasizes the value of a comprehensive strategy that includes dietary supplements.

Addressing any vitamin deficits that may emerge owing to the nature of the disease or dietary constraints is one of the main goals of adding supplements. Vasculitis can affect the body's ability to absorb and use nutrients, which can result in vitamin and mineral deficits that are essential for tissue regeneration and immune system function. As a result, supplements are a useful addition to diet plans, guaranteeing that the body gets the nutrients it needs to be in peak condition.

In addition, vitamins are essential for controlling inflammation, which is a defining feature of pancolitis. Some supplements include anti-inflammatory qualities that can help control the immune system and lessen the intensity of symptoms.

Healthcare providers can customize supplement regimens to meet individual demands by knowing the unique needs of individuals with Vasculitis. This helps to promote overall well-being.

It is important to remember that supplements are essential parts of a holistic care strategy for vasculitis and should not be used as stand-alone treatments. When combined with a thoughtfully planned diet, prescription drugs, and lifestyle adjustments, supplements help create a comprehensive strategy that addresses all facets of the illness.

Suggested Supplements for Individuals with Vasculitis:

For newcomers, navigating the world of supplements for vasculitis can be intimidating, but the process can be made simpler with a methodical and informed approach. Certain essential vitamins have demonstrated the potential to help people with Vasculitis on their path to better health, even if individual needs may differ.

1. Omega-3 Fatty Acids: Because of their strong anti-inflammatory qualities, omega-3 fatty acids are one of the main nutritional supplements for people with vasculitis. Fish and flaxseed oils are rich sources of these important fatty acids. Those who are new to taking supplements can simply add omega-3s to their regimen by choosing flaxseed oil or premium fish oil capsules. By controlling the inflammatory response, these nutrients may be able to lessen the symptoms of vasculitis.

2. Vitamin D: Since vitamin D regulates the immune system, it is an important dietary supplement for those with vasculitis.

Although vitamin D is naturally found in sunlight, supplements can be a trustworthy substitute, particularly for people who don't get much sun exposure. Novices can choose to use vitamin D3 supplements, as long as they follow doctor's recommendations and get the recommended daily dosage.

3. Probiotics: The role of gut health in immune function is becoming more widely acknowledged. Supplements containing probiotics, which are high in good bacteria, can help maintain a balanced gut microbiota. Beginners may choose from a range of foods high in probiotics or probiotic pills that contain strains of Lactobacillus and Bifidobacterium. In individuals with vasculitis, maintaining a balanced gut flora may help improve immune control.

4. Supplements containing turmeric or curcumin, which are well-known for their anti-inflammatory qualities, can be a beneficial addition to a food plan for those with vasculitis. Beginners can use turmeric in their food or locate these supplements in tablet form. To improve absorption, it is imperative to confirm if the supplement contains piperine or black pepper extract.

5. Multivitamins: A well-formulated multivitamin might be a convenient supplement for patients with Vasculitis to address potential nutrient shortages. Novices should select a multivitamin based on their unique requirements, taking into account elements like age, gender, and personal health state. This offers a thorough method for fulfilling the needs for important nutrients.

Therefore, dietary decisions and the supplements that are advised for patients with vasculitis work together to improve the overall management of the illness. Novices can start this adventure by speaking with medical experts to develop a customized supplement regimen that fits their unique requirements and preferences. This cooperative and supervised method guarantees an easy-to-use but efficient supplementation of the Vasculitis diet, enhancing health and life quality.

CHAPTER ELEVEN

LIFESTYLE TIPS FOR VASCULITIS MANAGEMENT

Exercise Recommendations:

Those who manage vasculitis must lead an active lifestyle since frequent exercise has a favorable effect on general health and well-being. But it's important to approach exercise cautiously and customize it to each person's ability. People with vasculitis should speak with their healthcare physician before beginning any exercise program to make sure the exercises they choose are safe and appropriate for their particular condition.

Low-impact exercise is a fantastic place to start for beginners. Excellent options that are easy on the joints and beneficial to the heart are cycling, walking, and swimming. Short sessions should be started, and as tolerance grows, the length should be gradually increased. Think about collaborating with a physical therapist or fitness expert who can design a customized workout program that takes into consideration the person's physical capabilities and any restrictions related to vasculitis.

It's crucial to combine strength and flexibility training with cardio workouts. Stretching exercises can lessen stiffness that is frequently linked to vasculitis and increase joint mobility. Every day, you can execute basic stretches for your main muscle groups to progressively increase your range of motion. Using resistance bands or small weights during strength training improves general physical function by toning muscles.

When starting an exercise regimen, consistency is essential. Aim for at least 150 minutes a week of moderate-intensity exercise while creating your realistic program. For beginners, this can be more doable if broken down into smaller, more manageable sessions. Pay attention to your body's needs and modify the time and intensity accordingly. Frequent exercise not only improves cardiovascular health but also aids in stress reduction, which is important for managing vasculitis.

Techniques for Stress Management:

For those who have vasculitis, stress management is essential since it can worsen symptoms and affect general health. Those who suffer from this illness can greatly improve their quality of life by putting stress management practices into practice. A simple and helpful technique is mindfulness meditation, which encourages relaxation and lowers tension by keeping an eye on the here and now.

Short meditation sessions can be easier for beginners to start with. Locate a peaceful, cozy area, take a seat or lie down, and close your eyes. Start by paying attention to your breathing and taking calm, deliberate breaths. As you get more accustomed to the exercise, gradually increase the time. There are numerous guided meditation apps and videos that offer beginners step-by-step instructions.

Another practical method for managing stress is to incorporate deep breathing exercises into everyday routines. When you practice diaphragmatic breathing, you take a deep breath via your nose, let your abdomen expand, and then gently release the breath through pursed lips. This method aids in triggering the body's relaxation response, which lowers tension and fosters serenity.

Taking part in enjoyable and relaxing activities is crucial for managing stress. Engaging in pleasurable activities such as gardening, reading, music listening, or socializing with loved ones can serve as a pleasant diversion from the difficulties associated with vasculitis. For beginners, finding activities that truly speak to them is essential to making sure they are sustainable and provide long-lasting stress reduction.

Creating a support network can also help manage stress. Making connections with people who are aware of the difficulties associated with vasculitis can offer emotional support and a sense of belonging. Getting counseling or joining support groups can provide insightful information and helpful coping mechanisms.

It takes time to learn how to prioritize self-care and incorporate stress management strategies into daily life, therefore beginners are urged to try out different approaches to see which one(s) suits them the best.

CHAPTER TWELVE

TRACKING AND MODIFYING YOUR NUTRITION

Recording Your Food:

The careful keeping of a food diary is one of the cornerstones of monitoring and modifying your diet in the context of cardiovascular disease. By taking a proactive stance, you can better understand your eating behaviors and identify potential triggers or trends that could aggravate your vasculitis symptoms.

Start by purchasing a special notebook or making use of a computer program made just for recording food consumption. Make categories, such as breakfast, lunch, supper, and snacks, on each page or section. Make columns to note the time of consumption, the amount consumed, any accompanying symptoms, and any changes in your overall health state in addition to this.

Maintaining consistency is essential. Try keeping a food journal of everything you eat, including drinks, sauces, and snacks. Remember to record the time of administration of any drugs or supplements you take. Having access to this comprehensive information helps medical professionals identify possible dietary triggers during consultations.

Starting this process could seem daunting to a newcomer. Simplify by concentrating on a single day at first, then progressively expanding the practice. Make notes on your phone or create a habit, such as taking notes after every meal. With time, you'll build a routine that helps you keep an eye on your diet and gives you valuable information to help you make changes based on sound judgment.

Frequent Consultations with Medical Experts:

Consultations with medical professionals frequently are essential while attempting to manage vasculitis with diet changes. These professionals—which include general practitioners, dietitians, and rheumatologists—offer professional advice customized to your particular situation, guaranteeing a comprehensive approach to your well-being.

Start by making an appointment schedule that you can stick to. These routine check-ins give medical staff the chance to keep an eye on your general health, evaluate the effects of dietary modifications, and modify your treatment plan as needed. During these sessions, it's important to communicate, so be ready to talk about your food diary, any symptoms you've seen, and any difficulties you're having following dietary advice.

It's critical to actively communicate with your healthcare team if you're new to the healthcare system. To make the most of your time with these experts, prepare a list of questions or concerns before each visit. Never be afraid to ask questions about dietary suggestions and to share any challenges you have following advice.

If you would like additional assistance during these check-ins, think about bringing along a family member or trusted friend.

During conversations regarding your health, they can support you emotionally, give fresh insights, and aid with memory. Frequent consultations foster a cooperative atmosphere that enables newcomers to actively engage in managing their vasculitis under the direction of experienced medical specialists.

CHAPTER THIRTEEN

INSPIRATIONS AND SUCCESS STORIES

Real-Life Accounts Of People Who Have Controlled Their Vasculitis With Diet:

Exploring the remarkable achievements of people who have controlled their Vasculitis with a diet that is specially designed for them presents a range of experiences characterized by tenacity, dedication, and life-changing dietary decisions. These tales offer hope and useful advice to people coping with the difficulties of venous insufficiency.

Introducing Sarah, a vibrant person who underwent a significant nutritional overhaul after being diagnosed with Vasculitis. She started her journey by speaking with a registered nutritionist who specialized in autoimmune disorders as well as an experienced healthcare provider. Together, they developed a specialized diet plan for people with Vasculitis that emphasized nutrient-dense foods and anti-inflammatory ones. Sarah saw her symptoms significantly improve over time with regular following to this approach. Her experience demonstrates the critical need for expert advice and a customized food plan in the successful management of vasculitis.

Another powerful story is that of James, who, after struggling with the difficulties of Vasculitis, discovered comfort and control in following an anti-inflammatory diet. Throughout his journey, he gradually switched from processed to whole, unprocessed foods. James's overall well-being and inflammation markers significantly decreased after he made fruits, vegetables, lean meats, and omega-3-rich diets his top priorities. His narrative emphasizes how altering one's diet to include particular foods can significantly reduce the symptoms of Vasculitis.

These first-hand reports highlight how crucial a customized nutrition plan is for managing ulcerative diabetes. Although every journey is different, a commitment to a thoughtful diet plan and cooperation with medical specialists run across these accounts, providing a path for those looking for motivation and direction.

Inspirational Advice On Maintaining A Healthy Lifestyle:

Starting a journey toward a lifestyle that is friendly to people with Vasculitis demands both steadfast motivation and a solid understanding of dietary guidelines. Maintaining a healthy lifestyle is a constant process that calls for both practical methods and mental toughness. Here, we look at inspirational advice to empower people in their pursuit of ideal health:

First and foremost, it's critical to have a specific, attainable goal. A clear objective provides direction, whether it's reaching a particular weight, lowering inflammatory markers, or improving general well-being. Divide more ambitious goals into more manageable benchmarks, and acknowledge each tiny victory as it occurs. This strengthens devotion to the path and gives a sense of accomplishment.

A key component of long-term adherence to the Vasculitis diet is including variation. To make meals interesting and fulfilling, try experimenting with a wide variety of fruits, vegetables, lean proteins, and complete grains. To make grocery shopping and meal preparation more doable for people, especially those who are unfamiliar with the dietary changes required by vasculitis, think about developing a weekly meal plan.

Creating a network of allies can greatly increase motivation. Through online forums, support groups, or local get-togethers, establish connections with people going through comparable experiences. It is reassuring to know that one is not traveling alone when one hears others talk about their experiences, advice, and victories.

When navigating the ups and downs of controlling Vasculitis with food, adopting an optimistic outlook is essential. Concentrate on any improvement that has been accomplished, no matter how tiny, and develop an appreciation for the body's resiliency. Deep breathing exercises and other mindfulness techniques can support a balanced mental attitude, which will help the lifestyle adjustments be more successful overall.

And last, adaptability is essential. Acknowledge that there might occasionally be setbacks or detours from the original plan on the path. Consider these experiences as teaching opportunities rather than failures. The capacity for both adaptation and course correction is essential to a viable and inspiring approach to a lifestyle that is favorable to people with Vasculitis.

Therefore, these inspirational ideas provide as a thorough road map for people managing their vasculitis and making their way toward a healthy lifestyle. Through the combination of a well-defined objective, a diverse diet, a network of supportive people, an optimistic outlook, and adaptability, people can develop the perseverance and determination required to make permanent progress on their health journey.

SUMMARY OF MAIN POINTS:

Through our investigation of the Vasculitis Diet Cookbook, we have gained a thorough grasp of the dietary needs of those who are afflicted with vasculitis, a collection of conditions marked by vascular inflammation. The cookbook is an invaluable tool for anyone controlling symptoms of vasculitis with thoughtful dietary selections. It provides a selection of recipes. This cookbook has outlined a process for creating dishes that are both delicious and compliant with vasculitis-friendly guidelines by combining nutritional science and creative cooking techniques.

Anti-inflammatory foods are important; this cookbook emphasizes this as one of its core concepts. These include whole grains, fish, nuts, and seeds, as well as fruits and vegetables high in antioxidants and omega-3 fatty acids. The focus on these ingredients comes from their ability to reduce inflammation, which is important for controlling the symptoms of vasculitis. The cookbook makes it easy for people to incorporate these food groups into their regular meals by giving a thorough explanation of each one.

The Vasculitis Diet Cookbook also emphasizes how important it is to keep a varied and well-balanced diet. It acknowledges that there isn't a single food or nutrient that can be the panacea for treating vasculitis, so it promotes a varied diet. This improves the enjoyment and sustainability of eating while also guaranteeing a wide range of vital nutrients. The cookbook painstakingly arranges recipes based on the various dietary requirements, which facilitates users in creating well-rounded meal plans.

The cookbook's attention to possible trigger foods is one of its most notable features. It considers the possibility that particular triggers may worsen symptoms in people with vasculitis. The cookbook gives its users the power to make educated decisions by clearly outlining which foods to limit or stay away from. For those who may not be familiar with the nuances of managing vasculitis through diet, this knowledge is essential.

Encouragement To Stick To A Diet That Is Favorable To Vasculitis:

More than just a recipe book, The Vasculitis Diet Cookbook is a helpful manual for anyone struggling to follow a diet that is appropriate for their type of vasculitis. Understanding that making dietary adjustments can be daunting, particularly for beginners, the cookbook provides helpful advice and suggestions to promote a healthy and long-lasting relationship with food.

First of all, the cookbook stresses the value of making changes gradually. It recognizes that implementing a new dietary strategy can be intimidating, particularly for people who are not familiar with the subtleties of managing vasculitis. To ensure a seamless transition, the cookbook recommends introducing modifications gradually. This could be experimenting with one or two vasculitis-friendly ingredients at a time, or introducing new recipes into weekly meal plans gradually.

People can adjust to the dietary recommendations without feeling overwhelmed if they take small, manageable steps.

Apart from the incremental method, the cookbook offers inspiring perspectives on the possible advantages of a diet suitable for people with vasculitis. It clarifies how specific foods can support both symptom management and general well-being. Users are more likely to remain motivated and dedicated to following the recommended guidelines if they are aware of the benefits of the food choices they make. This motivation is woven throughout the cookbook's story, supporting the notion that every meal made from its recipes is a proactive move in the direction of improved health.

The Vasculitis Diet Cookbook also promotes the idea of deviating from the rules when necessary. It acknowledges that life is dynamic and that following a strict diet can present difficulties. The cookbook makes sure that people can modify the recipes to fit their tastes and situations by providing workable answers and substitutes.

This adaptability is essential for long-term success because it keeps the diet from becoming a stressful endeavor and encourages a more long-term strategy for eating healthily.

Additionally, the cookbook incorporates inspirational success stories and testimonies from people who have effectively adopted a diet-friendly to people with vasculitis. This personal touch is inspirational because it shows that managing vasculitis through diet is not only possible but can also result in major improvements in quality of life when done with commitment and a positive outlook. For those who are just starting on their diet, these success stories serve as a source of encouragement and concrete proof that making a healthy change is possible.

As a result, the Vasculitis Diet Cookbook not only provides people with useful recipes but also gives them the confidence and motivation to embrace a diet that is friendly to their condition. Its all-encompassing approach guarantees that even beginners can easily navigate this culinary journey, resulting in optimal satisfaction and health outcomes. It does this by explaining important dietary principles and offering encouragement for sustained commitment.

MY GRATITUDES

Dear Valued Readers and Supporters,

I hope this message finds you well. I am writing to express my deepest gratitude to both God and each one of you for the overwhelming support and positive response to my book. Your encouragement and enthusiasm have truly touched my heart, and I am immensely thankful for the journey we are on together.

I believe that every success is a result of collaboration and support from various sources. First and foremost, I want to acknowledge the divine guidance and inspiration that led me to create this cookbook. Without the grace of God, this endeavor would not have been possible.

To my cherished readers, your commitment to exploring healthier dietary options for managing your crises has been both inspiring and humbling. Your trust in this book" means the world to me, and I am honored to be part of your journey toward improved health and well-being.

Also, I am reaching out to kindly request your valuable feedback on this book. Your thoughts and insights are crucial in helping me enhance and serve you better, ensuring that it continues to meet your needs effectively. Please take a moment to share your thoughts by rating and writing reviews on platforms where the book is available.

Your reviews not only provide me with invaluable feedback but also play a significant role in assisting others in making informed choices. By sharing your experiences, you contribute to a community that values health and wellness, creating a positive impact on countless lives.

Additionally, I encourage you to share this book with your friends, family and loved ones. Together, we can extend the reach of this promising resource, offering support and guidance to those who may benefit from it. Having this knowledge and seeking medical advice from your specialist I anticipate a turnaround for us.

Once again, thank you from the depths of my heart for your unwavering support. I am committed to continually improving and serving you better. Let us continue this journey together, promoting health, well-being, and a shared sense of community.

With sincere appreciation,

[Emmy Brooks]

Author, "VASCULITIS DIET COOKBOOK"

www.ingramcontent.com/pod-product-compliance
Lightning Source LLC
Chambersburg PA
CBHW070932290526

45795CB00001B/495